The Hepatology Compendium

Your Essential Guide to Mastering Liver Health and Disease Management

Tammy R. Sharp, DNP
Liver Health Specialist

Copyright © 2024 by Tammy R. Sharp, DNP
All rights reserved. No part of this publication may be reproduced, distributed, or transmitted in any form or by any means, including photocopying, recording, or other electronic or mechanical methods, without the prior written permission of the author, except in the case of brief quotations embodied in critical reviews and certain other noncommercial uses permitted by copyright law.

Acknowledgments

This book represents the culmination of years of dedication to the study and management of liver health, and I am profoundly grateful to those who supported me along this journey.

First and foremost, I would like to express my deepest gratitude to my patients, whose courage and resilience have been my greatest inspiration. Their experiences have shaped my understanding and fueled my passion for advancing liver health.

To my colleagues and mentors in hepatology, thank you for your guidance, encouragement, and the invaluable knowledge you have shared. Your contributions to the field and your commitment to improving patient care have been a driving force behind this work.

I am especially grateful to my family and friends for their unwavering support and patience during the long hours spent researching and writing. Your belief in me has been my anchor throughout this process.

Finally, I extend my appreciation to all healthcare providers who work tirelessly to improve liver health and the quality of life for their patients. This book is dedicated to you and the vital work you do every day.

With gratitude,
Tammy R. Sharp, DNP

Preface

Liver disease has become one of the leading causes of morbidity and mortality globally. Conditions such as chronic liver disease, non-alcoholic fatty liver disease (NAFLD), viral hepatitis, and cirrhosis affect millions, and these figures continue to rise each year. Despite this, liver health often does not receive the attention it deserves, both in clinical settings and public discourse. This book, The Hepatology Compendium: Your Essential Guide to Mastering Liver Health and Disease Management, aims to bridge that gap by providing a comprehensive, up-to-date, and clinically relevant resource for healthcare providers at every level.

As a Liver Health Specialist, I have dedicated my career to understanding the complexities of liver diseases and finding effective ways to improve patient outcomes. In my years of practice and research, it has become increasingly clear that knowledge alone is not enough to fight the growing epidemic of liver-related conditions. The integration of clinical expertise with evidence-based management strategies is essential in providing the best care for our patients.

This compendium is designed with both the novice and seasoned healthcare provider in mind. Whether you are a primary care physician, a specialist, a nurse practitioner, or a medical student, this book will serve as an essential tool in your daily practice. It is structured to provide you with the foundational knowledge of liver anatomy, physiology, and pathology, as well as practical, real-world applications for diagnosis and treatment.

In addition to covering a wide range of liver diseases, The Hepatology Compendium offers strategies for prevention and early detection, emphasizing the importance of early intervention to mitigate the impact of liver-related conditions.

As research into liver health evolves, so too does the understanding of how lifestyle factors—such as diet, exercise, and alcohol consumption—play a significant role in maintaining liver function and preventing disease. This book includes practical advice on these factors, alongside advanced therapeutic options that reflect the latest research in hepatology.

Throughout this work, I have included clinical case studies, diagnostic algorithms, and management strategies drawn from my years of clinical experience. My goal is not just to provide theoretical knowledge but to equip you with practical insights that you can implement in your practice immediately. I want this book to be a reference that you can turn to when facing the complexities of liver disease, whether in the office, the hospital, or in specialized care settings.

At its core, this book is about improving patient outcomes. Liver diseases, especially those diagnosed at advanced stages, have a profound impact on patients' lives. As healthcare professionals, it is our responsibility to provide patients with the best care, not just when they are sick, but in preventing illness and promoting wellness. This compendium is not just a tool for managing liver disease; it is a call to action for all of us to be proactive in our approach to liver health.

As you read through the chapters, I encourage you to reflect on how you can integrate the strategies and insights provided into your own practice. My hope is that this book will empower you to take a more active role in the management of liver health, and in doing so, improve the lives of countless patients.

I am deeply grateful for the opportunity to share my knowledge and experience with you. This book is a culmination of years of dedication to the field of hepatology, and it is my sincerest wish that it helps you achieve a deeper understanding of liver health and disease management.

Tammy R. Sharp, DNP
Liver Health Specialist

Foreword

The liver, a vital organ responsible for numerous essential functions, often remains underestimated in the realm of healthcare. It is the silent workhorse of the body, detoxifying blood, storing nutrients, and producing bile, among other tasks. Despite its critical importance, liver health is frequently overlooked, and the prevalence of liver disease continues to rise globally. In The Hepatology Compendium: Your Essential Guide to Mastering Liver Health and Disease Management, Dr. Tammy R. Sharp addresses this gap with profound expertise, offering an essential resource for healthcare professionals and those seeking to deepen their understanding of liver health.

Dr. Sharp, a seasoned Liver Health Specialist, brings a wealth of knowledge and experience to this comprehensive guide. Her approach is both practical and evidence-based, making complex hepatology concepts accessible while providing the tools necessary for managing a wide range of liver diseases. Throughout this book, readers will find a clear and structured examination of liver disease pathophysiology, diagnostic techniques, and treatment strategies. From the nuances of liver function to the management of diseases such as cirrhosis, hepatitis, and fatty liver disease, this compendium provides the clinical insights needed to optimize patient care and outcomes.

What sets this book apart is its ability to translate advanced hepatology concepts into practical, actionable information. It is an invaluable tool not only for healthcare professionals but also for those with an interest in liver health. Whether you are a medical student, practicing physician, nurse, or clinician, this book offers a well-rounded foundation to improve both knowledge and patient care.

Dr. Sharp's dedication to advancing the understanding of liver health is evident in every chapter. She writes with a passion for improving patient outcomes and empowering healthcare providers with the knowledge necessary to make informed decisions. Her expertise shines through as she delivers content that is both academically rigorous and clinically relevant.

As we continue to face an increasing global burden of liver disease, resources like this are more crucial than ever. The Hepatology Compendium serves as a beacon of knowledge, offering clarity and direction to those committed to mastering liver health and disease management.

I am confident that this book will not only enhance your understanding of hepatology but will also serve as a trusted companion in your professional journey. I highly recommend it to all those seeking to deepen their expertise in liver health and to make a tangible impact in the lives of their patients.

With sincere appreciation for Dr. Sharp's work, I am proud to endorse this important contribution to the field of hepatology.

Robert L. Brown, MD, Ph.D
Senior Clinical Researcher & Hepatology Specialist
Mayo Clinic
2024

Table of Contents

Common Hepatobiliary Presentations

1. Jaundice Evaluation
Structured Approach to History-Taking
Physical Examination
Investigative Steps
Unconjugated Hyperbilirubinemia
Conjugated Hyperbilirubinemia

2. Specific Clinical Scenarios
Biliary Pain with Normal Ultrasound
Dilated Common Bile Duct (CBD)
Dilated Intrahepatic Ducts with Normal CBD

3. Abnormal Liver Enzymes
Outpatient Context
Inpatient Context

4. Variceal Hemorrhage
Portal Hypertension and Management

5. Ascites
Initial Confirmation and Imaging
Fluid Analysis
Etiological Classification

6. Liver Lesions
Detected via Routine Ultrasound
Further Evaluation

7. Acute Liver Disease
Management Principles
Acute Liver Failure (ALF)
Referral for Liver Transplantation

8. Investigative Approach for Acute Liver Disease
Categories & Key Investigations

9. Management Overview
Generic Management
Specific Management for Paracetamol Overdose

10. Prognostication in Liver Injury

Hepatocellular Injury
Cholestatic Injury

11. Chronic Liver Disease & Hepatic Decompensation
Overview of Hepatic Decompensation
Management of Decompensation

Cirrhosis and Chronic Liver Disease Surveillance

1. Introduction to Chronic Liver Disease (CLD)
Overview of CLD Causes and Progression
Key Challenges in Diagnosis and Treatment

2. Hepatocellular Carcinoma (HCC) Surveillance
Screening Recommendations
Management

3. Variceal Surveillance
Screening and Management

4. Osteoporosis Surveillance
Risk Assessment and DEXA Scan Recommendations

5. Immunization Protocols
Vaccination Recommendations

6. Complications in Chronic Liver Disease
Encephalopathy, Malnutrition, and Variceal Hemorrhage

7. Endoscopic Management of Varices
EVL and Sclerotherapy

8. Key Causes of Chronic Liver Disease
Alcohol-Related Liver Disease (ALD)
Non-Alcoholic Steatohepatitis (NASH)
Hepatitis C Virus (HCV)

9. Management of Alcoholic Hepatitis

10. Hepatitis B Virus (HBV)
Transmission, Prevalence, and Management

11. Special Considerations in HBV
Pregnancy Management and Prophylactic Antiviral Therapy

12. Diagnosis and Management of Primary Biliary Cholangitis (PBC)

13. Diagnosis and Management of Primary Sclerosing Cholangitis (PSC)

14. Granulomatous Hepatitis
Etiologies and Treatment

15. Comprehensive Approach to CLD Management
Importance of Accurate Diagnosis and Integrated Care

Hereditary Liver Disorders

1. Hereditary Hemochromatosis
Overview, Diagnosis, and Management

2. Alpha-1 Antitrypsin Deficiency (A1ATD)
Overview, Diagnosis, and Management

3. Wilson's Disease
Clinical Features, Diagnosis, and Management

Liver Lesions and Hepatic Cancers

1. Hepatocellular Carcinoma (HCC)
Diagnosis, Staging, and Management

2. Hepatic Adenoma
Diagnosis and Management

3. Hepatic Haemangioma
Management

4. Focal Nodular Hyperplasia (FNH)
Management

5. Liver Metastases
Management

6. Liver Abscesses
Management

7. Liver Cysts
Management

Biliary and Pancreatic Diseases

1. Primary Sclerosing Cholangitis
Detailed Information

2. Chronic Pancreatitis
Diagnosis and Management

3. Autoimmune Pancreatitis and
IgG4-Associated Cholangitis
Diagnosis and Management

4. Pancreatic Adenocarcinoma
Diagnosis and Management

Liver Cancer: Management and Staging
Overview

1. Hepatocellular Carcinoma (HCC)
Staging and Treatment Modalities

2. Cholangiocarcinoma
Diagnosis, Staging, and Treatment Strategies

Introduction

The liver is a cornerstone of human health, influencing nearly every aspect of metabolic function, detoxification, and homeostasis. Yet, liver diseases remain a significant and often under-recognized challenge in modern medicine. Whether from viral infections, alcohol consumption, metabolic disorders, or genetic factors, liver conditions span a wide range of severity and complexity, often leading to irreversible damage if not managed appropriately. The need for a comprehensive, structured approach to liver disease diagnosis, treatment, and long-term management has never been more critical.

The Hepatology Compendium: Your Essential Guide to Mastering Liver Health and Disease Management is designed to meet this need, providing healthcare professionals with a thorough, evidence-based resource to navigate the complexities of liver health. Authored by Tammy R. Sharp, DNP, a seasoned expert in liver disease management, this book presents a detailed and practical guide to understanding and treating the full spectrum of hepatobiliary disorders. Drawing on years of clinical experience and the latest advancements in hepatology, this compendium ensures that practitioners are equipped with the knowledge required for optimal patient care.

The structure of this book offers a clear, logical framework that covers all critical aspects of liver health. From understanding basic hepatobiliary presentations, such as jaundice and abnormal liver enzymes, to the management of advanced liver diseases like cirrhosis, hepatocellular carcinoma, and hepatic decompensation, each chapter serves as both an educational tool and a practical guide. The comprehensive approach extends beyond traditional hepatology to incorporate aspects of hereditary liver disorders, liver cancer, and biliary and pancreatic diseases, offering clinicians a holistic understanding of liver-related conditions.

The content within The Hepatology Compendium is tailored for healthcare providers across a wide range of specialties, from general practitioners to hepatologists, offering in-depth insights into the nuances of diagnosing and managing liver diseases. By focusing on diagnostic clarity, evidence-based management strategies, and an understanding of the underlying pathophysiology, this book empowers clinicians to make informed decisions that will ultimately improve patient outcomes.

With its clear clinical guidelines, management algorithms, and diagnostic approaches, this compendium offers a structured framework for liver disease management. Special emphasis is placed on emerging trends and the latest advancements in hepatology, ensuring that readers are not only informed about current practices but also about cutting-edge approaches in the treatment of liver disorders.

The Hepatology Compendium aims to be a go-to reference for clinicians, students, and healthcare professionals, enhancing their understanding of liver health and offering them practical tools to address the challenges of liver disease management. By providing a comprehensive, accessible resource, this book strives to promote excellence in clinical care and improve the quality of life for individuals affected by liver conditions worldwide.

This guide is intended to be a trusted resource, enhancing both clinical practice and patient care, and ultimately contributing to the advancement of hepatology as a discipline.

Common Hepatobiliary Presentations

Jaundice

Effective evaluation of jaundice requires a structured approach. History-taking should focus on significant aspects such as:

Past medical history.

Drug usage (including recent prescriptions like co-amoxiclav or flucloxacillin).

Travel history, sexual activity, and use of illicit substances.

Symptoms such as pain and constitutional changes.

Physical examination may uncover signs of malignancy or localized tenderness suggestive of gallstone disease.

Initial Steps in Investigation:

1. Unconjugated Hyperbilirubinemia:

If painless jaundice is observed without cancer suspicion, unconjugated hyperbilirubinemia should be ruled out first.

Test split bilirubin levels to assess whether indirect bilirubin is disproportionately elevated.

Common diagnoses include haemolysis or conjugation defects like Gilbert's Syndrome.

2. Conjugated Hyperbilirubinemia:

Perform an ultrasound with Doppler studies to identify liver lesions or features of chronic liver disease.

In cases of normal ultrasound findings without pain or causative drugs, further evaluation involves screening for acute and chronic liver conditions.

Consider a biopsy for definitive diagnosis or prognosis if initial tests are inconclusive.

Specific Clinical Scenarios:

Biliary Pain with Normal Ultrasound: Likely choledocholithiasis, which requires imaging of the biliary tree via MRCP or EUS to confirm before performing ERCP.

Dilated Common Bile Duct (CBD): Most often caused by CBD stones or pancreatic cancer.

Stones detected on ultrasound should be managed with ERCP.

For suspected malignancies, perform a staging CT and EUS with biopsy.

Dilated Intrahepatic Ducts with Normal CBD: Differential diagnoses include cholangiocarcinoma, primary or secondary sclerosing cholangitis, or extrinsic compression (e.g., metastases). Advanced imaging with MRCP or dynamic MRI is recommended.

Abnormal Liver Enzymes

Elevated liver enzymes are a frequent reason for both inpatient and outpatient referrals.

1. Outpatient Context:

History and examination should assess for chronic liver disease, biliary pathologies, hereditary conditions, and risk factors.

Initial investigations should evaluate:

Disease severity: PT, albumin, bilirubin.

Chronic liver disease markers: Platelets, Fibroscan, biopsy.

Cause identification: Liver screen, Doppler ultrasound.

2. Inpatient Context:

Causes include acute liver disease, chronic liver disease, or secondary phenomena (e.g., drug reactions, ischemia, malignancy).

Acute liver failure and decompensated liver disease require urgent identification due to high morbidity and mortality.

Variceal Hemorrhage

Portal hypertension may first manifest as variceal bleeding. Immediate treatment involves resuscitation and endoscopic therapy while investigating the underlying cause, typically cirrhosis or venous thrombosis. An ultrasound with Doppler studies is a critical initial test.

Ascites

Ascites is a common presentation requiring systematic evaluation:

1. Initial Confirmation and Imaging:

Confirm ascites with ultrasound and obtain a triple-phase CT scan.

Perform an ultrasound-guided tap to analyze fluid.

2. Fluid Analysis:

Tests include protein concentration, SAAG (serum-ascites albumin gradient), cell counts, and microbiology.

3. Etiological Classification:

Exudative Ascites (e.g., peritonitis, malignancy, TB).

Transudative Ascites (e.g., portal hypertension, heart failure).

Liver Lesions

Liver lesions are often detected during routine ultrasound screening. Further evaluation typically involves:

Tumor markers and imaging (triphasic CT, MRI).

Biopsy guided by MDT decisions for diagnosis and staging.

Proper staging and management strategies depend on lesion type, patient history, and clinical findings.

Acute Liver Disease

Acute liver disease refers to a rapid onset of liver dysfunction. It does not include decompensated chronic liver disease (often termed acute-on-chronic liver failure).

Management Principles

The management of acute liver disease involves:

1. Identification: Recognize liver impairment (non-vitamin K-dependent coagulopathy) or liver failure (characterized by coagulopathy and encephalopathy).

2. Diagnosis: Establish the underlying cause.

3. Treatment: Provide generic and condition-specific interventions.

4. Monitoring: Tailor the level of monitoring to the severity of the liver injury:

Inpatient care for significant jaundice or liver impairment.

Outpatient care with frequent follow-ups for less severe cases.

Although most cases of acute liver injury do not progress to acute liver failure, the latter is addressed first due to its significant mortality risk.

Acute Liver Failure (ALF)

Acute liver failure is classified based on the time from jaundice onset to the development of hepatic encephalopathy:

Hyperacute: Encephalopathy occurs within 7 days.

Acute: Encephalopathy develops in 1–5 weeks.

Subacute: Encephalopathy develops in 5–26 weeks.

Prognosis:

Hyperacute ALF: Better outcomes despite severe encephalopathy and coagulopathy.

Acute ALF: Moderate prognosis.

Subacute ALF: Poor prognosis with higher mortality, though cerebral edema and coagulopathy are less pronounced.

Referral for Liver Transplantation:

Patients suspected of developing ALF should be promptly referred to a transplant center unless contraindicated. Advanced encephalopathy (grades 3–4) requires ventilation during transfer to mitigate cerebral edema risk.

Indications for Liver Transplantation in ALF

1. Paracetamol Poisoning:

pH < 7.25 after 24 hours with fluid resuscitation.

Coagulopathy (PT > 100 seconds or INR > 6.5), serum creatinine > 300 μmol/L or anuria, and grade 3–4 encephalopathy.

Serum lactate > 3.5 mmol/L on admission or > 3.0 mmol/L after fluid resuscitation.

2. Non-Paracetamol Causes (e.g., Hepatitis A, B, Seronegative Hepatitis, Drug Reactions):

Coagulopathy (PT > 100 seconds or INR > 6.5) with any encephalopathy grade.

Any encephalopathy grade plus three of the following: unfavorable etiology, age > 40 years, jaundice-to-encephalopathy time > 7 days, bilirubin > 300 μmol/L, or PT > 50 seconds (INR > 3.5).

3. Wilson's Disease:

Coagulopathy and any grade of encephalopathy.

Investigative Approach for Acute Liver Disease

Category	Key Investigations
Viral Hepatitis	Viral exposure History, IgM for HAV, HBc, HEV, EBV, Serology
Drugs/Toxins	Exposure history, Drug levels, eosinophil count
Autoimmune Hepatitis	ANA. SMA, LKM, antibodies , IgG levels
Wilson's Disease	Serum copper, ceruloplasmin, hemolysis markers, Layser-fleischer rings, ALP levels
Malignancy	Imaging histology
Pregnancy-related	Ultrasound, uric acid, HELLP evaluation

| Ischemic Hepatitis | History of hypotension/sepsis, Arterial embolism risk factors |

Management Overview

Generic Management:

1. Metabolic Corrections: Address glucose, potassium, phosphate, and sodium imbalances.

2. Coagulopathy: Do not correct unless bleeding is evident; thrombocytopenia is addressed only when bleeding occurs.

3. Sepsis Prophylaxis: Use antibiotics (e.g.,) and antifungals (e.g., fluconazole).

4. Hemodynamic Support: Ensure fluid resuscitation and transfusion as needed.

Specific Management for Paracetamol Overdose:

Administer N-acetylcysteine (NAC):

150 mg/kg in 200 mL 5% glucose over 15 minutes.

50 mg/kg in 500 mL 5% glucose over 4 hours.

100 mg/kg in 1000 mL 5% glucose over 16 hours.

Continue NAC until paracetamol levels are undetectable and PT is < 20 seconds.

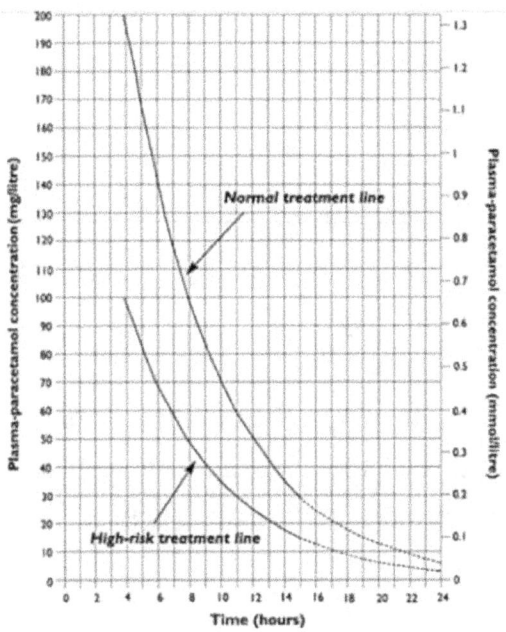

Fig. 1 Treatment Protocols for Paracetamol Poisoning: Dosing Curves for NAC Administration

Other Drug-Induced Liver Injuries:

Evaluate carefully for immune-mediated or non-immune drug reactions.

Cease offending drugs and monitor progress.

Prognostication

Hepatocellular Injury: ALT > 3x ULN and bilirubin > 2x ULN indicate a poor prognosis (10–15% mortality).

Cholestatic Injury: Prognosis improves after discontinuing the offending drug unless vanishing bile duct syndrome is present.

Early identification, comprehensive monitoring, and timely referral to specialized centers are essential for optimal outcomes in acute liver disease.

Chronic Liver Disease and Hepatic Decompensation: A Comprehensive Overview

Hepatic decompensation is a late-stage manifestation of liver disease, as the liver has remarkable compensatory capacity, often requiring only 20% of hepatocytes to function effectively. Decompensation can be either acute or chronic in nature. Acute chronic decompensation results from an additional insult, such as sepsis, medication, toxins, metabolic imbalances, constipation, or secondary liver damage from alcohol or viral hepatitis. Other factors like hepatocellular carcinoma (HCC) or portal vein thrombosis due to altered portal circulation can also contribute. Chronic decompensation, however, is a direct consequence of the underlying liver pathology.

Decompensation refers to the liver's failure to maintain normal physiological functions, which can be classified into synthetic, metabolic, immunological, and haemodynamic functions. It is crucial to identify the cause of decompensation, assess these functions, and address each accordingly. While normalizing these functions may not always be feasible, management focuses on slowing disease progression, with liver transplantation or death being eventual outcomes in advanced cases.

1. Synthetic Function

The liver's synthetic function is evaluated by the production of albumin and clotting factors. While correcting these factors in the chronic setting is generally unnecessary, if bleeding complications arise, the administration of fresh frozen plasma (FFP), cryoprecipitate, and possibly platelets may be beneficial. In cases of sepsis, particularly spontaneous bacterial peritonitis (SBP), albumin infusion has been shown to be helpful.

2. Metabolic Function

Metabolic function is assessed through nutritional status, the presence of encephalopathy, and serum bilirubin levels.

Nutritional support is vital in both acute and chronic stages, and osteoporosis screening and management are essential in long-term care. Treatment often includes calcium and vitamin D supplementation.

3. Immunological Function

Liver disease typically results in compromised immune function, leading to frequent infections. Patients with decompensated chronic liver disease should be considered immunosuppressed for several reasons: the liver's failure to clear antigens from the portal circulation, metabolic disruptions affecting immune cell function, and a lack of production of key immune components like complement and albumin. Once a systemic infection occurs, acute hepatic decompensation often follows, exacerbating immune dysfunction and perpetuating a cycle of infection and liver failure. Prompt use of broad-spectrum antibiotics is essential until a causative organism is identified.

4. Haemodynamic Function

Haemodynamic decompensation is typically progressive, following the peripheral vasodilation hypothesis. Key stages include cirrhosis, portal hypertension, and splanchnic vasodilation, which leads to reduced effective arterial blood volume. This activates vasoconstrictor systems and induces renal vasoconstriction, ultimately resulting in systemic hypotension, ascites, and hyponatremia. In severe cases, hepatorenal syndrome (HRS) develops. Management of these complications includes managing ascites, monitoring blood pressure, and treating renal dysfunction.

Cirrhosis and Chronic Liver Disease Surveillance

1. Hepatocellular Carcinoma (HCC) Surveillance

Patients at risk for HCC should undergo regular screening, including a six-month ultrasound and serum AFP testing. High-risk groups include all cirrhotic patients, men over 40, women over 50, and African patients with HBV. If a lesion greater than 1 cm or elevated AFP is found, further imaging with MRI should be performed. If AFP is normal and lesions are under 1 cm, follow-up with ultrasound every 3 months is recommended. Management of HCC is individualized and discussed in multidisciplinary teams.

2. Variceal Surveillance

Cirrhotic patients should be enrolled in a variceal screening program. Follow-up endoscopies are scheduled based on the presence of varices and the degree of liver disease. Management decisions for small, medium, and large varices, including beta-blockers or endoscopic variceal band ligation (EVL), depend on the risk of bleeding. Banding is performed at intervals until eradication is achieved, followed by regular surveillance.

3. Osteoporosis Surveillance

Patients with cirrhosis, particularly those with primary biliary cirrhosis (PBC), primary sclerosing cholangitis (PSC), or those on long-term steroids, should be assessed for osteoporosis. This includes calcium and vitamin D supplementation, and dual-energy X-ray absorptiometry (DEXA) scans every 3–5 years. Treatment for osteoporosis involves bisphosphonates or hormone replacement therapy for females with hypogonadism.

4. Immunization Protocols

Patients with chronic liver disease, especially those with hepatitis C or cirrhosis of any etiology, should be vaccinated against hepatitis A and B. Pneumococcal and annual influenza vaccines are also recommended.

Complications in Chronic Liver Disease

1. Encephalopathy

The diagnosis of hepatic encephalopathy is challenging and typically involves clinical assessment, ammonia testing, and possibly EEG. Encephalopathy is graded from mild confusion (Grade 1) to coma (Grade 4). Treatment of acute encephalopathy includes optimizing liver perfusion, managing bowel function with lactulose, and avoiding hepatically metabolized sedatives. Chronic encephalopathy may require lactulose, rifaximin, and potentially liver transplantation if resistant.

2. Malnutrition

Malnutrition is a common issue in decompensated cirrhosis. Outpatient management involves encouraging small, frequent meals, with nutritional supplementation. In inpatient settings, severe malnutrition may necessitate nasogastric feeding.

3. Variceal Hemorrhage

Variceal hemorrhage requires immediate resuscitation, correction of blood abnormalities (such as anemia, thrombocytopenia, and coagulopathy), and empirical broad-spectrum antibiotics. Vasoconstrictors like terlipressin or octreotide are used prior to endoscopy, which should ideally occur within 4 hours. If hemorrhage cannot be controlled, a TIPS (transjugular intrahepatic portosystemic shunt) or surgical intervention may be necessary. Endoscopic variceal band ligation (EVL) or injection sclerotherapy are primary treatment modalities for varices.

Endoscopic Management

EVL is the preferred treatment for bleeding esophageal and cardiac varices. If EVL fails, sclerotherapy using ethanolamine or histoacryl glue can be considered. Regular follow-up endoscopies are required for ongoing management of varices.

Chronic liver disease (CLD) encompasses a range of conditions characterized by progressive liver damage. In the UK, the leading causes are alcohol-related liver disease (ALD), non-alcoholic steatohepatitis (NASH), and hepatitis C virus (HCV). Accurate diagnosis requires comprehensive liver screening for all CLD patients. Misdiagnoses are common, and many patients present with multiple contributing factors, potentially impacting treatment decisions and transplant eligibility. A structured approach is critical to ensure proper diagnosis and management.

Key Causes of Chronic Liver Disease

1. Alcohol-Related Liver Disease (ALD):
ALD is the most prevalent form of liver disease in clinical practice, largely due to excessive alcohol consumption. Its impact varies among individuals due to genetic predisposition, comorbidities (e.g., obesity, HCV), and gender. ALD manifests in four primary forms:

Fatty liver (reversible with abstinence).

Alcoholic hepatitis (acute inflammation with jaundice).

Chronic liver disease with cirrhosis.

Hepatocellular carcinoma (HCC).

Management:

Abstinence is paramount and can result in significant liver recovery within two years. Support systems, such as the Norwich Recovery Partnership, are essential.

Pharmacological interventions like acamprosate and baclofen may assist in maintaining sobriety.

Severe cases of alcoholic hepatitis are evaluated using the Maddrey Discriminant Function (DF). Patients with DF > 32 have a high mortality risk, necessitating corticosteroid therapy (e.g., prednisolone 40 mg daily for one month, barring contraindications). Pentoxifylline may be an alternative, especially for renal-compromised patients.

2. Non-Alcoholic Steatohepatitis (NASH):

NASH is a spectrum of liver conditions associated with metabolic syndrome, obesity, and diabetes. It can progress to cirrhosis and HCC. Diagnosis relies on imaging and biopsy findings of steatosis and inflammation.

3. Hepatitis C Virus (HCV):
HCV is a significant contributor to chronic liver inflammation and fibrosis. Modern antiviral therapies (e.g., direct-acting antivirals) have transformed HCV management, achieving high cure rates.

Screening: Anti-HCV antibody tests, followed by RNA quantification and genotyping, guide treatment decisions.

Management: Early treatment prevents cirrhosis, liver failure, and HCC.

Alcoholic Hepatitis

Alcoholic hepatitis presents as jaundice, malaise, and liver dysfunction. Histologically, it is characterized by steatohepatitis, neutrophilic infiltration, and cholestasis. Differentiation from sepsis is critical as the clinical presentation often overlaps.

Prognostic Assessment:
The Maddrey Discriminant Function (DF) stratified risk:

DF > 32: High mortality risk; consider corticosteroids or pentoxifylline.

DF < 32: Favorable prognosis; supportive care suffices.

Treatment Guidelines:

Supportive measures, including fluid management, avoidance of diuretics, nutritional support, and vitamin supplementation, are essential.

Corticosteroids improve short-term survival but require careful monitoring for infection.

Hepatitis B Virus (HBV)

Transmission and Prevalence:
HBV is transmitted through blood and bodily fluids. Approximately 2% of the UK population is affected by HBV or HCV.

Natural History:

1. Acute Clearance: Over 95% of immunocompetent adults clear HBV, but this decreases significantly in childhood infections.

2. Chronic HBV (CHB): Patients progress through distinct phases:

Immune Tolerance: High viral replication without liver damage.

Immune Reactive: Immune-mediated liver damage occurs, necessitating monitoring of ALT and HBV DNA levels. Treatment includes pegylated interferon (finite) or tenofovir (lifelong).

Inactive Carrier State: Low viral replication with minimal liver damage. Close monitoring is required to detect reactivation.

HBsAg Negative Phase: Seroclearance occurs, marking disease resolution.

Management Strategies:

Regular monitoring (e.g., ALT, HBV DNA) and biopsy when indicated.

First-line antiviral therapy: Tenofovir 245 mg daily, with monitoring for renal function and potential side effects.

Hepatocellular carcinoma (HCC) surveillance for high-risk groups.

Immunization of contacts and newborns to prevent transmission.

Special Considerations:

Pregnancy: Tenofovir is safe and prevents vertical transmission.

Immunosuppression: Prophylactic antiviral therapy is essential to prevent HBV reactivation in patients undergoing chemotherapy or immunosuppressive treatment.

Clinical Insights and Recommendations

1. Accurate Diagnosis: Comprehensive liver panels ensure correct identification of CLD etiology.

2. Biopsy and Imaging: Elastography and biopsy provide critical insights into liver fibrosis and inflammation, guiding treatment.

3. Integrated Care: Collaboration with multidisciplinary teams, including addiction services and metabolic specialists, optimizes outcomes.

Comprehensive Overview and Detailed Analysis of Hepatobiliary Disorders

Primary Biliary Cholangitis (PBC)

PBC is a chronic liver disease predominantly affecting women, with a female-to-male ratio of nearly 10:1. It commonly presents in middle age and is characterized by progressive destruction of intrahepatic bile ducts.

Diagnosis:

Serology: The hallmark diagnostic markers are anti-mitochondrial antibodies (AMA) and anti-pyruvate dehydrogenase (anti-PDH) antibodies, with over 95% specificity and 98% sensitivity. In AMA-negative cases, further antibody testing (e.g., through Cambridge immunology laboratories) may be necessary.

Biochemical Indicators: Elevated alkaline phosphatase (ALP) and γ-glutamyl transpeptidase (GGT) levels (≥2× upper limit of normal) are characteristic findings. Liver biopsy is reserved for atypical presentations.

Clinical Features:

Symptoms include fatigue, pruritus, and lethargy. Osteoporosis and hyperlipidemia are also common, with the latter not significantly increasing atherosclerosis risk.

Prognosis: Disease progression varies; younger patients at diagnosis and those failing to meet Paris II criteria (bilirubin >1× ULN, ALT >2× ULN, and ALP >3× ULN after one year of ursodeoxycholic acid therapy) typically have a worse prognosis. The Mayo PBC Score aids in advanced-stage prognostication.

Management:

First-Line Therapy: Ursodeoxycholic acid (12-15 mg/kg) slows disease progression and alleviates pruritus.

Refractory Cases: Alternatives include budesonide for significant hepatitis, fenofibrate, and symptomatic treatments such as cholestyramine, rifampicin, naltrexone, ondansetron, or extracorporeal albumin dialysis (MARS).

Surveillance: Ultrasound assessments for portal hypertension and hepatocellular carcinoma (HCC) screening are recommended biannually.

Patients with bilirubin >50 μmol/L should be evaluated for liver transplantation.

Primary Sclerosing Cholangitis (PSC)

PSC is strongly linked to inflammatory bowel disease (IBD) and negatively associated with smoking. Unlike PBC, PSC affects both intrahepatic and extrahepatic bile ducts.

Diagnosis:

Imaging: Magnetic resonance cholangiopancreatography (MRCP) is the diagnostic modality of choice. Endoscopic retrograde cholangiopancreatography (ERCP) is reserved for therapeutic interventions.

Biomarkers: Perinuclear antineutrophil cytoplasmic antibodies (pANCA) have a sensitivity of 70% and specificity of 90%.

Liver Biopsy: Utilized for disease staging, although transient elastography's role remains under investigation.

Management:

IBD Screening: Colonoscopy at diagnosis and regular surveillance in PSC-IBD patients to detect neoplasia.

Medical Therapy: Ursodeoxycholic acid (15-18 mg/kg) may reduce pruritus and cholangiocarcinoma risk, but discontinuation is advised in non-responders.

Complications: Treat dominant strictures with stenting or dilation and manage recurrent cholangitis with antibiotics.

Surveillance for Cholangiocarcinoma:
Annual imaging (ultrasound and MRCP) and CA 19-9 testing, though the latter has limited specificity. Gallbladder polyps warrant cholecystectomy.

PSC exhibits variable phenotypes. Intrahepatic PSC often has a more benign course, especially in women. Median survival post-diagnosis ranges from 20-25 years.

Granulomatous Hepatitis

The primary etiologies include PBC, sarcoidosis, and drug reactions. Diagnosis involves clinical evaluation and targeted investigations:

Sarcoidosis: High-resolution CT, pulmonary function tests, and transbronchial biopsy.

Drugs: Comprehensive medication history and literature review.

Infectious Causes: Mycobacterial cultures, viral PCRs, and antibody titers (e.g., Q fever, brucellosis).

Management:

Sarcoidosis treatment includes prednisolone tapered to maintenance doses (10-15 mg/day) over six months, supplemented by steroid-sparing agents like azathioprine or mycophenolate as needed.

Hereditary Hemochromatosis

An autosomal recessive disorder caused by HFE gene mutations (C282Y and H63D), leading to systemic iron overload. Women are typically protected until menopause due to menstruation.

Diagnosis:

Ferritin >200 μg/L and transferrin saturation >50% are diagnostic markers.

Genetic testing for HFE mutations confirms the diagnosis. Liver biopsy is warranted for cirrhosis assessment.

Management:

Venesection is the mainstay of therapy, initiated weekly and spaced out as ferritin normalizes (<50 μg/L). Maintenance therapy occurs every 2-4 months.

Screen first-degree relatives for genetic mutations and iron overload.

Alpha-1 Antitrypsin Deficiency (A1ATD)

A1ATD results from mutations in the SERPINA1 gene, most commonly the Z and S alleles.

Diagnosis:

Serum A1AT levels <1 g/L warrant phenotypic analysis.

Liver biopsy shows characteristic A1AT accumulation.

Management:

There is no definitive treatment. Risk factor mitigation (e.g., avoidance of alcohol and smoking) is critical. Screen first-degree relatives for A1ATD variants.

Wilson's Disease

An autosomal recessive disorder of copper metabolism caused by mutations in the ATP7B gene. This results in copper accumulation in the liver, brain, and other tissues.

Clinical Features:

Presentations range from hepatic (e.g., cirrhosis, acute liver failure) to neurological (e.g., dystonia, parkinsonism) and psychiatric symptoms.

Diagnosis:

Key investigations include slit lamp examination for Kayser-Fleischer rings, ceruloplasmin levels, and 24-hour urinary copper excretion. Liver biopsy confirms elevated hepatic copper content (>250 μg/g).

Management:

Chelation therapy with agents like penicillamine or trientine. Zinc supplementation inhibits copper absorption.

Public Health Focus: Addressing lifestyle factors like alcohol consumption and obesity is crucial to reducing CLD prevalence.

Liver Lesions

Hepatocellular Carcinoma (HCC)

Hepatocellular carcinoma (HCC) typically arises in the context of cirrhosis, making it essential to rule out cirrhosis in any patient presenting with HCC.

Diagnosis

When a new nodule measuring ≤1 cm is detected during surveillance ultrasound, repeat imaging is advised at three months to differentiate between cirrhotic nodules and HCC. For lesions >1 cm, classical imaging features such as arterial enhancement and portal venous washout confirm diagnosis. These characteristics result from hypervascularity coupled with the absence of portal venous blood supply. In cases where classical imaging features are absent, additional cross-sectional imaging is recommended. If results remain inconclusive, biopsy may be performed, though this is generally avoided due to the risk of tumor seeding. Measurement of alpha-fetoprotein (AFP) serves as an adjunct diagnostic tool.

Staging and Management

The Barcelona Clinic Liver Cancer (BCLC) staging system integrates tumor stage, liver disease severity, and performance status (PS) to guide treatment strategies. Management options include:

Surgery or Ablation: Suitable for patients with resectable lesions and compensated liver disease.

Liver Transplantation (OLT): Offered to patients meeting transplant criteria, with radiofrequency ablation (RFA) or transarterial chemoembolization (TACE) as bridging therapies.

Non-Curative Options: For patients ineligible for transplantation or surgery, TACE or systemic therapy (e.g., sorafenib) is recommended. Patients with advanced liver dysfunction (Child-Pugh C) or poor PS are limited to supportive care.

Extended Transplantation Criteria (UK):

Single tumor ≤5 cm.

Up to five tumors ≤3 cm.

Single tumor >5 cm but ≤7 cm, with stable disease (≤20% volume increase) over six months, no vascular invasion, and AFP <100,000.

Hepatic Adenoma

Hepatic adenomas are benign tumors, often solitary, and associated with combined oral contraceptives (COCP), anabolic steroids, or metabolic conditions like glycogen storage disorders (GSD) and MODY type 3.

Diagnosis

Initial detection is typically via ultrasound, showing hyperechoic lesions. CT imaging reveals well-demarcated, isodense (or hyperdense in fatty liver) lesions that enhance during the arterial phase. MRI findings include high signal intensity on T2-weighted images and arterial enhancement after gadolinium. Lesion biopsy may be needed for definitive diagnosis, especially in atypical presentations.

Management

Discontinue COCP or anabolic steroids.

Consider surgical resection for lesions >5 cm due to potential malignancy.

Monitor non-resected lesions annually using ultrasound/MRI and AFP levels.

Pregnant patients require close monitoring at 4 and 8 months via ultrasound.

Hepatic Haemangioma

Haemangiomas are the most common benign liver tumors, predominantly affecting women aged 30–50 years. They are often asymptomatic but can cause pressure symptoms or complications such as rupture or high-output cardiac failure if large.

Radiological Features

Ultrasound: Hyper-reflective lesion.

CT: Hypodense mass with nodular peripheral enhancement and centripetal filling on delayed phases.

MRI: Smooth, well-demarcated mass hyperintense on T2-weighted images with progressive enhancement ("filling-in") during delayed imaging.

Management

Asymptomatic lesions <2 cm require no further investigation. Larger or symptomatic haemangiomas may necessitate resection.

Conservative management is appropriate in most cases.

Focal Nodular Hyperplasia (FNH)

FNH is a common benign lesion, often incidentally detected in women aged 20–50 years. It is thought to result from a hyperplastic response to anomalous arterial perfusion.

Radiological Features

Ultrasound: Variable appearance; central scar visible in 20% of cases.

CT: Hypodense/isodense lesion on non-contrast images, becoming hyperdense during arterial phase with potential central scar enhancement.

MRI: High signal intensity of the scar on T2-weighted images; rapid enhancement with gadolinium.

Management

Conservative management is appropriate when imaging is characteristic. Lesional biopsy may be considered if diagnosis remains uncertain. Rarely, resection is performed for pain attributable to FNH.

Liver Metastases

Liver metastases often present as multiple hypoechoic lesions on ultrasound. Their characteristics on CT or MRI depend on the primary tumor. For example, colorectal metastases appear hypodense, while vascular tumors (e.g., neuroendocrine) are hyperintense.

Management

Management focuses on identifying and addressing the primary malignancy. Liver biopsy is often diagnostic in cases where the primary tumor remains unidentified.

Liver Abscesses

Liver abscesses, often caused by infections originating in the biliary tree or bowel, present with fever and localized pain.

Management

Initiate intravenous antibiotics (e.g.,).

Abscesses <3 cm: Antibiotics alone with weekly imaging.

Abscesses 3–5 cm: Consider aspiration alongside antibiotics.

Abscesses >5 cm: Percutaneous drainage with IV and oral antibiotics.

Amoebic abscesses, common in travelers, are treated with oral metronidazole (500–750 mg three times daily for 7–10 days).

Liver Cysts

Simple Cysts: These asymptomatic lesions are usually incidental findings and require no intervention unless symptomatic. Large cysts may necessitate deroofing or resection for complications like infection or rupture.

Polycystic Liver Disease: Congenital liver disorders causing abdominal mass sensation and pain. Management focuses on symptomatic relief and acute care of complications.

Hepatic Cystadenoma: Rare, potentially malignant cystic lesions requiring resection.

Biliary and Pancreatic Diseases: A Comprehensive Overview

Primary Sclerosing Cholangitis

(Refer to the above for detailed information.)

Chronic Pancreatitis

Chronic pancreatitis is characterized by prolonged inflammation that leads to architectural remodeling, fibrosis, and calcifications in the pancreas. Key clinical manifestations include persistent abdominal pain, diarrhea, unintentional weight loss, and diabetes mellitus symptoms. Some individuals may present with complications such as pseudocysts, ductal obstructions, or splenic vein thrombosis.

Diagnostic Approach

The diagnosis relies heavily on imaging modalities (e.g., CT, MRCP) and identification of secondary complications like exocrine pancreatic insufficiency (diagnosed via low fecal elastase).

Risk Factors

Toxic or Metabolic: Alcohol abuse, tobacco use, medications, chronic renal failure, and hypocalcemia.

Genetic Mutations: Cationic trypsinogen gene (PRSS1 - autosomal dominant), CFTR, and SPINK1 (both autosomal recessive).

Autoimmune Etiologies: Includes autoimmune pancreatitis.

Recurrent/Obstructive: Recurrent acute pancreatitis, pancreatic divisum, neoplasms, or ductal obstructions caused by stones or external compression.

Management

Management focuses on eliminating the underlying cause and addressing complications:

1. Exocrine Deficiency: Presenting as steatorrhea and weight loss, treated with pancreatic enzyme replacement therapy (e.g., Creon).

2. Endocrine Deficiency: Managed with insulin therapy for glucose intolerance or diabetes.

3. Pain Control: Secondary causes like duct strictures or pseudocysts are managed surgically or endoscopically. For refractory pain, an analgesic regimen may be combined with interventions like celiac plexus neurolysis or pancreatic resections.

Complications such as pseudocyst drainage, strictures, and stones often necessitate specialist care. Surgical or endoscopic options are determined on a case-by-case basis.

Autoimmune Pancreatitis and IgG4-Associated Cholangitis

Autoimmune pancreatitis (AIP) typically manifests as abdominal pain or obstructive jaundice and may show radiological findings like pancreatic duct strictures or diffuse gland enlargement ("sausage-shaped pancreas").

Diagnostic Criteria

As per the Mayo Clinic guidelines:

1. Histological features on biopsy.

2. Imaging findings with elevated IgG4 (>2x upper limit of normal).

3. Elevated IgG4 levels alone with significant steroid responsiveness.

Treatment Protocol

Initial therapy involves prednisolone (30–40 mg daily for 2–4 weeks), tapered gradually.

In steroid-refractory cases, azathioprine (2 mg/kg/day) is recommended.

Prognostic factors include high baseline IgG4 levels and biliary strictures.

Associated Conditions

Type 1 AIP is often systemic, with associations such as inflammatory bowel disease, Sjögren's syndrome, retroperitoneal fibrosis, and tubulointerstitial nephritis. Type 2 AIP, typically linked to inflammatory bowel disease, often resolves with a single steroid course.

IgG4-Associated Cholangitis

This condition mimics primary sclerosing cholangitis (PSC) but demonstrates superior outcomes with appropriate steroid therapy. An elevated IgG4 level is pivotal in distinguishing it from PSC.

Pancreatic Adenocarcinoma

Pancreatic adenocarcinoma is a highly aggressive malignancy, often presenting with painless jaundice (tumors in the pancreatic head) or nonspecific symptoms like weight loss and abdominal pain.

Diagnosis and Staging

Diagnosis involves:

Imaging: Ultrasound followed by CT, with histological confirmation via endoscopic ultrasound (EUS)-guided fine-needle aspiration (FNA).

Staging: Based on the TNM classification.

Staging:

Primary Tumor (T): Extent of local spread (e.g., T1-T4).

Lymph Nodes (N): Presence of regional lymph node involvement.

Metastasis (M): Distant spread (e.g., M0, M1).

Treatment Modalities

1. Surgical Resection: Considered for localized disease without vascular invasion.

2. Chemotherapy: May be administered alone or adjunctively.

3. Radiotherapy: Used selectively for unresectable cases.

4. Palliative Care: Focuses on symptom relief through stenting, analgesia, or celiac plexus neurolysis.

Prognosis: Median survival is <6 months, with a five-year survival rate <5%.

Cholangiocarcinoma

Cholangiocarcinoma arises from the biliary epithelium and may be intrahepatic or ductal. Common presentations include jaundice or liver masses.

Diagnosis and Staging

Imaging: CT and MRI with MRCP provide essential diagnostic roadmaps.

Staging: Employs systems like the Bismuth or TNM classifications.

Treatment Strategies

1. Surgical Resection: The cornerstone of management in resectable cases, with procedures tailored to tumor location (e.g., Whipple's procedure for distal tumors).

2. Adjuvant Therapy: Limited evidence exists for chemotherapy or radiotherapy benefits but may be considered.

3. Palliation: Focused on biliary drainage and symptom relief in unresectable cases.

Prognosis: Five-year survival rates range from 5% to 40%, contingent on disease stage and resectability.

References

1. European Association for the Study of the Liver (EASL). Clinical Practice Guidelines for the Management of Chronic Liver Disease and Hepatocellular Carcinoma. Journal of Hepatology.

2. American Association for the Study of Liver Diseases (AASLD). Guidance on the Diagnosis, Management, and Treatment of Hepatic Conditions. Hepatology.

3. World Gastroenterology Organisation (WGO). Global Guidelines on Acute and Chronic Liver Disease. World Journal of Gastroenterology.

4. National Institute for Health and Care Excellence (NICE). Diagnostic and Management Protocols for Liver and Biliary Conditions. NICE Clinical Guidelines.

5. Schiff ER, Sorrell MF, Maddrey WC. Schiff's Diseases of the Liver. 12th ed. Wiley-Blackwell; 2017.

6. Boyer TD, Manns MP, Sanyal AJ, editors. Zakim and Boyer's Hepatology: A Textbook of Liver Disease. 7th ed. Elsevier; 2017.

7. Fauci AS, Kasper DL, Hauser SL, et al., editors. Harrison's Principles of Internal Medicine. 21st ed. McGraw-Hill Education; 2022.

8. Curry MP, Chopra S. Acute Liver Failure and Chronic Hepatic Conditions: Key Clinical Insights. The New England Journal of Medicine.

9. Dooley JS, Lok AS, Burroughs AK, Heathcote J. Sherlock's Diseases of the Liver and Biliary System. 13th ed. Wiley-Blackwell; 2018.

10. American College of Gastroenterology (ACG). Clinical Updates on Portal Hypertension

and Hepatic Encephalopathy. ACG Clinical Guidelines.

11. Centers for Disease Control and Prevention (CDC). Guidelines on Viral Hepatitis Surveillance and Management. CDC Viral Hepatitis Program.

12. National Institutes of Health (NIH). Liver Disease Research and Emerging Trends in Hepatology. NIH Research Publications.

13. Jalan R, Williams R. Liver Failure and Transplantation. Lancet Hepatology Series.

14. World Health Organization (WHO). WHO Guidelines on Hepatitis B and C Treatment. WHO Publications on Viral Hepatitis.

15. Roberts SK, Strasser SI. Management of Ascites and Portal Hypertension in Cirrhotic Patients. Journal of Gastroenterology and Hepatology.

16. Clinical Liver Disease (CLD) Journal. Special Issues on Hereditary Liver Disorders and Emerging Therapies.

17. Murray KF, Hadzic N. Pediatric Liver Disease: A Global Perspective. Pediatric Clinics of North America.

18. Institute of Liver Studies. Comprehensive Research on Wilson's Disease and Alpha-1 Antitrypsin Deficiency. King's College London Publications.

19. National Liver Foundation (NLF). Public Health Initiatives and Research on Non-Alcoholic Fatty Liver Disease (NAFLD).

20. Gastrointestinal Endoscopy Journal. Advances in Endoscopic Management of Biliary and Pancreatic Diseases.

Glossary

1. **Acute Liver Failure (ALF):** A rapid deterioration of liver function in a person without pre-existing liver disease, often associated with coagulopathy and encephalopathy.

2. **Alcoholic Hepatitis**: Inflammation and damage to the liver caused by excessive alcohol consumption, often associated with jaundice, ascites, and liver failure.

3. **Alpha-1 Antitrypsin Deficiency (A1ATD):** A hereditary disorder characterized by low levels of alpha-1 antitrypsin, leading to liver disease and lung issues such as emphysema.

4. **Ascites**: The accumulation of fluid in the peritoneal cavity, commonly due to portal hypertension from liver cirrhosis.

5. **Autoimmune Hepatitis (AIH):** A chronic liver disease where the immune system attacks liver cells, causing inflammation and potentially leading to fibrosis or cirrhosis.

6. **Biliary Atresia**: A rare pediatric condition in which the bile ducts are abnormally narrow or blocked, leading to liver damage and requiring early surgical intervention.

7. **Biliary Pain**: Discomfort originating from the bile ducts, often caused by obstruction or inflammation.

8. **Cholangiocarcinoma**: A rare type of cancer that occurs in the bile ducts, often presenting with jaundice and abdominal pain.

9. **Cholestasis**: A condition characterized by impaired bile flow, either within the liver (intrahepatic) or outside it (extrahepatic), resulting in jaundice and pruritus.

10. **Chronic Liver Disease (CLD):** Long-term liver damage that progresses over months or years, potentially leading to cirrhosis and hepatic decompensation.

11. **Cirrhosis**: A chronic liver disease characterized by scarring (fibrosis) and impaired liver function due to long-term damage from various causes, such as hepatitis or alcohol abuse.

12. **Conjugated Hyperbilirubinemia**: An increase in conjugated (direct) bilirubin in the blood, often indicating liver or biliary tract dysfunction.

13. **Endoscopic Variceal Ligation (EVL):** A therapeutic procedure used to manage esophageal varices by tying them off to prevent or control bleeding.

14. **FibroScan (Transient Elastography):** A non-invasive imaging technique used to assess liver stiffness and detect fibrosis or cirrhosis.

15. **Focal Nodular Hyperplasia (FNH)**: A benign liver lesion, often asymptomatic, that typically does not require treatment.

16. **Gilbert's Syndrome**: A genetic condition causing mild, intermittent unconjugated hyperbilirubinemia due to reduced activity of the enzyme UGT1A1.

17. **Hepatic Adenoma**: A rare, benign liver tumor often linked to oral contraceptive use or anabolic steroid use, with a risk of rupture or malignant transformation.

18. **Hepatic Encephalopathy**: A neuropsychiatric complication of liver dysfunction, resulting from the buildup of toxins like ammonia in the bloodstream.

19. **Hepatic Steatosis**: Commonly referred to as fatty liver, a condition where excess fat accumulates in liver cells, which may progress to NASH or cirrhosis.

20. **Hepatocellular Carcinoma (HCC)**: The most common primary liver cancer, often associated with chronic hepatitis or cirrhosis.

21. **Hepatorenal Syndrome (HRS):** A severe complication of advanced liver disease characterized by functional kidney failure due to reduced renal blood flow.

22. **Hereditary Hemochromatosis**: A genetic disorder causing excessive iron absorption, leading to iron overload in organs, including the liver.

23. **Hyperbilirubinemia**: Elevated levels of bilirubin in the blood, a hallmark of liver dysfunction or hemolysis, often manifesting as jaundice.

24. **IgG4-Associated Cholangitis**: A type of autoimmune cholangitis associated with elevated IgG4 levels, often seen with autoimmune pancreatitis.

25. **Jaundice**: Yellowing of the skin and eyes due to elevated bilirubin levels in the blood, often a symptom of liver or biliary disease.

26. **MELD Score (Model for End-Stage Liver Disease):** A scoring system used to assess the severity of chronic liver disease and prioritize liver transplant recipients.

27. **Non-Alcoholic Fatty Liver Disease (NAFLD):** A spectrum of liver conditions unrelated to alcohol consumption, ranging from simple steatosis to NASH.

28. **Non-Alcoholic Steatohepatitis (NASH):** An advanced form of non-alcoholic fatty liver disease (NAFLD) characterized by liver inflammation and damage.

29. **Paracetamol Overdose**: The most common cause of acute liver failure, resulting from the toxic metabolite NAPQI, which depletes glutathione reserves.

30. **Portal Hypertension**: Increased pressure within the portal venous system, often a consequence of cirrhosis, leading to complications like varices and ascites.

31. **Portal Vein Thrombosis (PVT)**: A blockage of the portal vein by a blood clot, often seen in cirrhosis or hypercoagulable states.

32. **Primary Biliary Cholangitis (PBC)**: A chronic autoimmune disease that damages bile ducts in the liver, leading to bile buildup and liver damage.

33. **Primary Sclerosing Cholangitis (PSC)**: A progressive disease causing scarring and narrowing of the bile ducts, often associated with inflammatory bowel disease.

34. **Pruritus**: A common symptom in liver diseases, especially in cholestatic conditions, caused by bile salt accumulation in the bloodstream.

35. **Regenerative Nodules**: Benign liver nodules formed as a response to liver injury, typically seen in cirrhosis, which can sometimes mimic liver tumors.

36. **Spontaneous Bacterial Peritonitis (SBP)**: A bacterial infection of ascitic fluid without an apparent source, commonly occurring in patients with cirrhosis.

37. **Steatohepatitis**: Inflammation of the liver due to fat accumulation, often leading to fibrosis and cirrhosis if left untreated.

38. **Unconjugated Hyperbilirubinemia**: Elevated levels of unconjugated (indirect) bilirubin in the blood, typically caused by excessive hemolysis or impaired bilirubin processing by the liver.

39. **Varices**: Enlarged veins, commonly in the esophagus or stomach, caused by portal

hypertension and prone to life-threatening bleeding.

40. **Wilson's Disease**: A rare hereditary condition leading to excessive copper accumulation in the liver, brain, and other organs, requiring lifelong treatment.

41. **Xanthelasma**: Yellowish deposits of cholesterol-rich material, often seen in patients with cholestatic liver diseases like PBC.

www.ingramcontent.com/pod-product-compliance
Lightning Source LLC
Chambersburg PA
CBHW050326230526
45471CB00005B/2364